The Fastest Keto Fat Bombs for Beginners

*The Complete Collection of Keto Fat Bombs and Candies –
Enjoy your Keto Diet*

Jessica Simpson

Contents

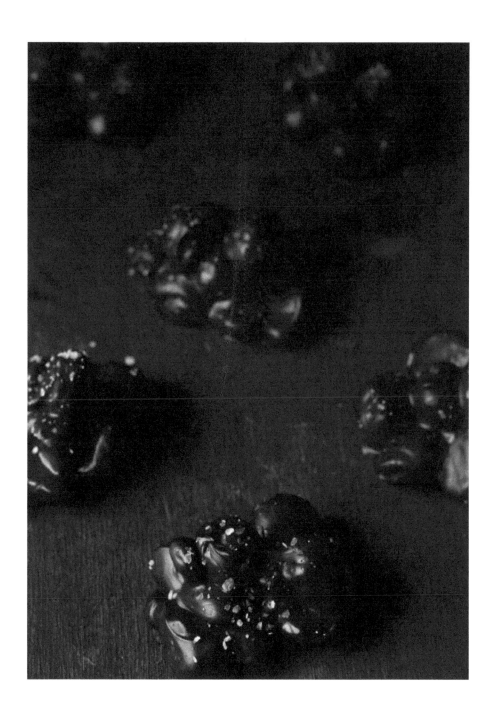

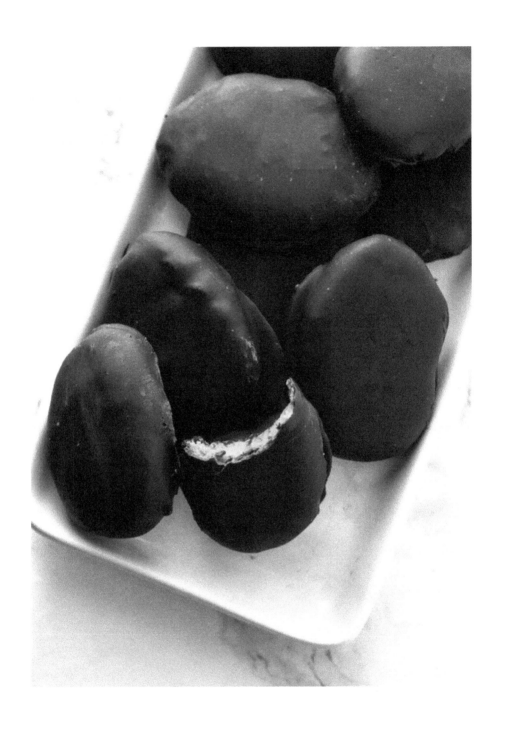

Keto Chocolate Kisses

Servings: 20

Cooking Time: 15 Minutes

Ingredients:

- 2 ounces unsweetened baking chocolate
- 1 ½ tablespoons Swerve confectioners' powdered sweetener
- ¼ teaspoon vanilla extract
- A pinch stevia concentrated powder
- ½ ounce food grade cocoa butter

Directions:

1. Add chocolate, sweetener and cocoa butter into a heatproof bowl.
2. Place the bowl in a double boiler. Stir occasionally until the mixture melts. You can also melt it in a small pan over low heat.
3. Add stevia and vanilla and mix well.
4. Spoon into 20 chocolate molds. Cool completely.
5. Chill until firm. Remove from mold and serve.
6. Leftovers can be stored in an airtight container in the refrigerator.

Nutrition Info: Per Servings: Calories: 24.8 kcal, Fat: 2.2 g, Carbohydrates: 0.8 g, Protein: 0.4 g

White Chocolate Fat Bombs

Servings: 8

Cooking Time: 0 Minute

Ingredients:

- 6 tablespoons cacao butter, melted
- 1 cup coconut cream
- 4 teaspoons vanilla essence
- 3 tablespoons College Latin
- Pinch of salt
- 1/2 cup water
- 3 tablespoons granulated swerve

Directions:

1. Dissolve gelatin in water in a small bowl and let it sit for 5 minutes.
2. Combine all the remaining ingredients in a saucepan on low heat while stirring.
3. Add gelatine and mix well until dissolved.
4. Divide the mixture into the silicone molds.
5. Refrigerate them for 1 hour.
6. Serve after removing them from the molds.

Nutrition Info: Per Servings: Calories 136 Total Fat 10.g Saturated Fat 0.5 g Cholesterol 4 mg Total Carbs 1.2 g Sugar 1.4 g Fiber 0 g Sodium 45 mg Potassium 31 mg Protein 0. g

Raspberry Fat Bombs

Servings: 12

Cooking Time: 0 Minutes

Ingredients:

- 1 cup coconut butter
- 1 cup of coconut milk
- ½ cup of coconut oil
- ¼ cup cacao butter
- 1 teaspoon vanilla essence
- ¼ cup freeze-dried raspberries
- Stevia to taste

Directions:

1. Place the paper liners in the muffin cups of a tray.
2. Cook everything in a saucepan for minutes on medium heat.
3. Mix well then allow it to cool for 5 minutes.
4. Divide the mixture into the muffin cups.
5. Place one raspberry on top of each muffin.
6. Then keep the muffin tray in the refrigerator for 3 hours.
7. Remove the fat bombs from the muffin cups.
8. Serve.

Nutrition Info: Calories 261 ;Total Fat 27.1 g ;Saturated Fat 23.4 g ;Cholesterol 0 mg ;Sodium 10 mg ;Total Carbs 6.1 g ;Sugar 2.1 g ;Fiber 3.g ;Protein 1.8 g

Peppermint Marshmallows

Servings: 8

Cooking Time: 20 Minutes

Ingredients:

- 1 cup water, divided
- 2 1/2 tbsp gelatine, grass fed
- 2/3 cup Swerve powder
- 1/8 tsp cream of tartar
- 2/3 cup Bocha Sweet
- Pinch salt
- 1 tsp peppermint extract

Directions:

1. Layer an 8-inch pan with parchment paper and grease it with cooking spray.
2. Mix half of the water-gelatin in a small bowl. Let it sit for 5 minutes.
3. Heat the remaining water with sweetener in a saucepan.
4. Add salt, gelatine, and cream of tartar. Mix well to dissolve the sweetener.
5. Cook the mixture to reach at 240 degrees F then turn off the heat.
6. Beat this hot syrup in a stand mixer on low speed until it thickens, for about 15 minutes.

7. Spread this mixture in a baking pan evenly.

8. Refrigerate it for 4 hours.

9. Break into pieces then serve.

Nutrition Info: Per Servings: Calories 76 Total Fat 7.2 g Saturated Fat 6.4 g Cholesterol 0 mg Total Carbs 2g Sugar 1 g Fiber 0.7 g Sodium 8 mg Potassium 88 mg Protein 2.2 g

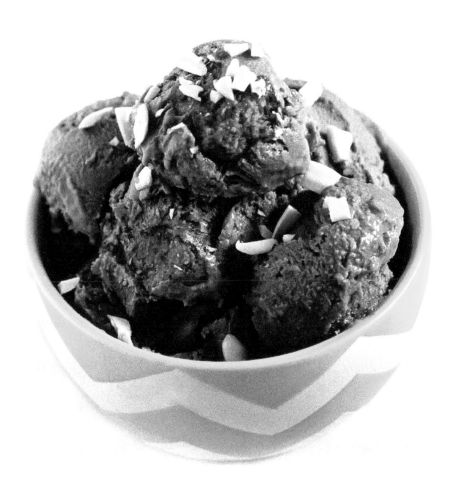

Cocoa Butter Candy

Servings: 8

Cooking Time: 5 Minutes

Ingredients:

- 14 cup cocoa butter
- 10 drops stevia
- 14 cup coconut oil

Directions:

1. Melt together coconut oil and cocoa butter in a saucepan over low heat.
2. Remove from heat and stir in stevia.
3. Pour mixture into the silicone candy mold and refrigerate until hardened.
4. Serve and enjoy.

Nutrition Info: Per Servings: Net Carbs: 0g; Calories: 119; Total Fat: 13.8g; Saturated Fat: 9.9g Protein: 0g; Carbs: 0g; Fiber: 0g; Sugar: 0g; Fat 100% Protein 0% Carbs 0%

Frozen Chocolate Roll

Servings: 8

Cooking Time: Na

Ingredients:

- 1 cup raw pecans
- 1 ounce unsweetened baking chocolate
- ½ tablespoon vanilla extract
- ½ cup grated or shredded coconut, unsweetened
- 1 ½ tablespoons Swerve or 2 teaspoons green stevia

Directions:

1. Add pecans, chocolate, vanilla, coconut and sweetener into the food processor bowl. Process until well incorporated.
2. Place a sheet of parchment paper on your countertop. Place the mixture on the parchment paper.
3. Roll into a log with the help of the parchment paper.
4. Wrap the log with parchment paper and freeze until firm.
5. Place on your cutting board. Unwrap and cut into ½ inch thick slices.
6. Serve immediately or transfer into a freezer safe container and freeze until use.

Nutrition Info: Per Servings: Calories: 144 kcal, Fat: 14 g, Carbohydrates: 4.35 g, Protein: 2 g

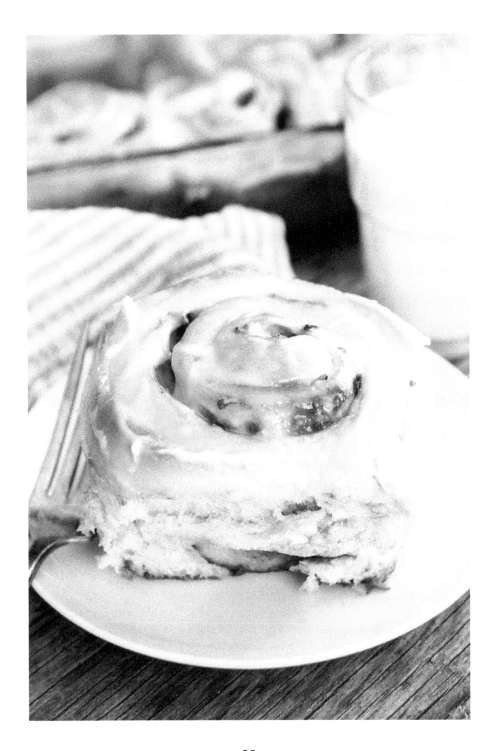

Keto Lemon Drop Gummies

Servings: 8

Cooking Time: 15 Minutes

Ingredients:

- ½ cup fresh lemon juice
- 4 tablespoons gelatin powder
- 2 tablespoons water
- 4 tablespoons erythritol or stevia to taste

Directions:

1. Add water and lemon juice into a saucepan. Place saucepan over low heat.
2. Add gelatin and erythritol and stir constantly it completely dissolved.
3. Pour into a cup or small jar with a spout.
4. Pour into gummy molds. Chill until it sets.
5. Remove from mold and serve.
6. Leftovers can be stored in an airtight container in the refrigerator. These can keep for 7 days.

Nutrition Info: Per Servings: Calories: 275 kcal, Fat: 0 g, Carbohydrates: 1.25 g, Protein: 6.1 g

Coconut Blueberry Gummies

Servings: 8

Cooking Time: 0 Minute

Ingredients:

- 2 cups of coconut milk
- A ¼ cup of blueberry juice
- ¼ cup gelatine, grass fed

Directions:

1. Mix gelatine with blueberry juice in a bowl.
2. Heat coconut milk in a saucepan over medium heat.
3. Whisk in gelatine mixture and stir cook until dissolved.
4. Remove the pan from the heat then divide the mixture into silicone molds.
5. Refrigerate them for 2 hours to set.
6. Serve after removing them from the molds.

Nutrition Info: Per Servings: Calories 200 Total Fat 21.1 g Saturated Fat 19.5 g Cholesterol 14.2 mg Total Carbs 1.1 g Sugar 1.3 g Fiber 0.4 g Sodium 46 mg Potassium 145 mg Protein 0.4 g

Low-carb Keto "andes" Candies

Servings: 8

Cooking Time: 15 Minutes

Ingredients:

- 1 ½ tablespoons coconut oil, melted
- 2 tablespoons coconut manna, melted
- 1 tablespoon Dutch process cocoa powder
- 1 ½ tablespoons Swerve confectioners' powder
- 1 tablespoon chocolate MCT oil powder
- 2-3 drops peppermint extract

Directions:

1. Add coconut oil, coconut manna and peppermint extract into a bowl and mix well.
2. Add cocoa, Swerve and oil powder into a bowl and stir. Add into the bowl of wet ingredients.
3. Pour into 8 fat bomb molds.
4. Chill until firm.
5. Remove from mold and serve.
6. Leftovers can be stored in an airtight container in the refrigerator. These can keep for 4 – 5 days.

Nutrition Info: Per Servings: Calories: 64 kcal, Fat: 6.125 g, Carbohydrates: 1.9 g, Protein: 0.6 g

Dark Chocolate Candy

Servings: 16

Cooking Time: 5 Minutes

Ingredients:

- 4 oz unsweetened dark chocolate
- 12 tsp vanilla
- 12 cup coconut oil
- 3 tbsp butter
- 12 cup walnut butter

Directions:

1. Melt coconut oil, butter, and dark chocolate in a saucepan over medium heat until smooth.
2. Remove from heat and stir in walnut butter and vanilla.
3. Pour mixture into the silicone candy mold and refrigerate until set.
4. Serve and enjoy.

Nutrition Info: Per Servings: Net Carbs: 1.4g; Calories: 177; Total Fat: 17.; Saturated Fat: 10.1g Protein: 2.2g; Carbs: 2.9g; Fiber: 1.5g; Sugar: 0.3g; Fat 89% Protein 6% Carbs 5%

Ginger Coconut Candy

Servings: 10

Cooking Time: 5 Minutes

Ingredients:

- 1 tsp ground ginger
- 14 cup shredded coconut, unsweetened
- 3 oz coconut oil, softened
- 3 oz coconut butter, softened
- 1 tsp liquid stevia

Directions:

1. Add coconut oil and coconut butter in a microwave-safe bowl and microwave for 30 seconds. Stir well.
2. Add remaining ingredients and stir well to combine.
3. Pour mixture into the silicone candy mold and refrigerate until hardened.
4. Serve and enjoy.

Nutrition Info: Per Servings: Net Carbs: 0.8g; Calories: 130 Total Fat: 13.9g; Saturated Fat: 12.1g Protein: 0.6g; Carbs: 2.3g; Fiber: 1.; Sugar: 0.6g; Fat 96% Protein 2% Carbs 2%

Lemon Lime Coconut Candy

Servings: 20

Cooking Time: 1 Hour And 10 Minutes

Ingredients:

- 1/2 cup shredded coconut, unsweetened
- 1 lemon, zested and juiced
- 2 limes, zested and juiced
- 1/8 teaspoon sea salt
- 1 teaspoon liquid stevia
- 1 teaspoon vanilla extract, unsweetened
- 1/4 teaspoon lemon extract, unsweetened
- 1/4 teaspoon lime extract, unsweetened
- 1 cup coconut butter
- 1/2 cup coconut oil

Directions:

1. Place a small saucepan over low heat, add coconut butter and oil and cook for 2 to 3 minutes or until melts.
2. Then whisk in remaining ingredients until smooth and spread the mixture into the glass dish.
3. Place dish into the freezer for 1 hour or until firm and then cut into chunks.
4. Serve straight away or store in the freezer.

Nutrition Info: Calories: 136 Cal, Carbs: 2 g, Fat: 13.7 g, Protein: 1 g, Fiber: 2 g.

Mexican Spiced Chocolate

Servings: 25-27

Cooking Time: 10-15 Minutes

Ingredients:

- ¾ cup cocoa powder
- ½ teaspoon ground cinnamon
- 1/8 teaspoon pepper powder
- ¾ teaspoon chili powder
- ¼ teaspoon ground nutmeg
- 1/8 teaspoon fine sea salt
- ½ teaspoon vanilla extract
- 2.5 ounces cacao butter
- 35-40 drops liquid stevia or monk fruit sweetener to taste

Directions:

1. Add all of the dry ingredients into a mixing bowl and stir.
2. Place a saucepan over low heat. Add the cacao butter into it. When it melts, turn off heat. You can also melt it in a double boiler.
3. Add vanilla and stevia into the saucepan and mix well. Pour into the bowl of dry ingredients and mix until well combined.

4. Pour into chocolate molds. Let the chocolate cool to room temperature. Refrigerate until they set.

5. Remove from the mold and serve.

6. Leftovers can be stored in an airtight container in the refrigerator. These can keep for 5-days.

Nutrition Info: Per Servings: Calories: 24 kcal, Fat: 3.3 g, Carbohydrates: 0.6 g, Protein: 0.5 g

Chocolate Kisses Candy

Servings: 12

Cooking Time: 0 Minute

Ingredients:

- 1 oz cocoa butter
- 1/2 teaspoon vanilla essence
- 4 oz sugar free baking chocolate
- 1/8 teaspoon stevia powder
- 3 tablespoons swerve powder

Directions:

1. Melt chocolate with cocoa butter and sweetener in a bowl by heating in a microwave.
2. Stir in vanilla essences and stevia and mix well.
3. Pour this mixture into candy molds.
4. Freeze the candies until set.
5. Serve after removing them from the molds.

Nutrition Info: Per Servings: Calories 2 Total Fat 27.1 g Saturated Fat 23.4 g Cholesterol 0 mg Total Carbs 6.1 g Sugar 2.1 g Fiber 3.9 g Sodium 10 mg Potassium 57 mg Protein 1.8 g

Hibiscus Gelatin Gummies

Servings: 4

Cooking Time: 5 Minutes

Ingredients:

- 1 3/4 cup hot water
- 3 passion tea bags
- 6 tablespoons grass fed gelatine

Directions:

1. Pour water in a saucepan and cook it to boil then turn off the heat.
2. Place the tea bags in hot water and steep them for 10 minutes.
3. Remove the tea bags from the water.
4. Mix gelatine powder in ½ cup of tea water.
5. Return the remaining tea water to the heat.
6. Let this water heat then stir in gelatine mixture.
7. Stir cook for 1 minute then divides the mixture into a candy mold tray.
8. Place this tray in the refrigerator for 1 hour.
9. Remove the candies from the molds.
10. Enjoy.

Nutrition Info: Calories 38 ;Total Fat 0.6 g ;Saturated Fat 0 g ;Cholesterol 0 mg ;Sodium 33 mg ;Total Carbs 0 g ;Sugar 0 g ;Fiber 0 g ;Protein 9 g

Chocolate Truffles

Servings: 12

Cooking Time: 2 Hours And 5 Minutes

Ingredients:

- 2 medium avocados, pitted and peeled
- 1/2 cup chopped pecans
- 1/2 cup cocoa powder, unsweetened
- 1 tablespoon swerve sweetener
- 2 tablespoons chocolate flavored syrup
- 2 tablespoons avocado oil
- 2 tablespoons heavy whipping cream

Directions:

1. Place all the ingredients except for pecans in a blender and pulse at high speed for to 2 minutes or until combined.
2. Tip the mixture in a bowl and chill in the refrigerator for 1 hour or more until firm.
3. Then shape the mixture into 12 balls, each about 1-inch in size, and roll in the pecans.
4. Return balls into the refrigerator and chill for 1 hour or until firm.
5. Serve straightaway.

Nutrition Info: Calories: 111 Cal, Carbs: 4.5 g, Fat: 10 g, Protein: 1.5 g, Fiber: 3 g.

Chocolate Coconut Candies

Servings: 20

Cooking Time: 55 Minutes

Ingredients:

- Coconut Candies:
- 3 tablespoons swerve sweetener
- 1/2 cup shredded coconut, unsweetened
- 1/2 cup coconut butter
- 1/2 cup avocado oil
- Chocolate Topping:
- 1-ounce chocolate, unsweetened
- 1/4 cup swerve sweetener
- 1/4 cup cocoa powder
- 1/4 teaspoon vanilla extract, unsweetened
- 1.5 ounces cocoa butter

Directions:

1. Line 20 mini muffin pans with paper liners and set aside.
2. Place a saucepan over low heat, add butter and oil and cook for 3 minutes or more until melted, stirring frequently.
3. Then stir in coconut and sweetener until combined and divide the mixture evenly between prepared muffin cups.

4. Place muffin cups into the freezer and chill for 30 minutes or more until firm.

5. In the meantime, prepare chocolate topping and for this, place butter and chocolate in a bowl and microwave for 4seconds or more until melted.

6. Stir well, add remaining ingredients for topping and stir until combined.

7. When candies are firm, remove from freezer and spoon prepared chocolate topping on them.

8. Let chocolate coated candies sit for 15 minutes at room temperature.

9. Serve straightaway.

Nutrition Info: Calories: 240 Cal, Carbs: 5 g, Fat: 25 g, Protein: 2 g, Fiber: 1 g.

Vanilla Fat Bombs

Servings: 25-28

Cooking Time: 10 Minutes

Ingredients:

- 2 cups unsalted macadamia nuts
- ½ cup coconut butter at room temperature
- ½ cup virgin coconut oil, at room temperature
- Seeds from 2 vanilla beans or 4 teaspoons sugar-free vanilla extract
- 4 tablespoons powdered erythritol or Swerve
- 20-30 drops liquid stevia (optional)

Directions:

1. Add macadamia nuts into a food processor. Set on medium speed. Process until smooth.
2. Transfer into a bowl. Add butter and coconut oil and mix well. If the butter and coconut oil is not soft, then melt in a double boiler.
3. Add erythritol, vanilla and stevia and mix well.
4. Spoon about 1-½ tablespoons of the mixture into each of the mini muffin molds or ice cube trays.
5. Chill until firm.
6. Remove from mold and serve.
7. Leftovers can be stored in an airtight container in the refrigerator. These can keep for 4 – 5 days.

Nutrition Info: per Servings: Calories: 137.kcal, Fat: 14.76 g, Carbohydrates: 2.52 g, Protein: 0.8 g

Chocolate Candy

Servings: 10

Cooking Time: 10 Minutes

Ingredients:

- ½ cup of coconut oil
- ½ cup unsweetened cocoa powder
- ½ cup almond butter
- 1 tbsp stevia
- ½ tbsp sea salt

Directions:

1. Melt coconut oil and almond butter in a saucepan and over medium heat.
2. Add cocoa powder and sweetener and stir well.
3. Remove pan from heat and let it cool for 5 minutes.
4. Pour saucepan mixture in silicone candy mold and place in the refrigerator for 15 minutes or until set.
5. Serve and enjoy.

Nutrition Info: Per Servings: Net Carbs: 1g; Calories: 109; Total Fat: 11.9g; Saturated Fat: 9.8g Protein: 1g; Carbs: 2.5g; Fiber: 1.5g; Sugar: 0.1g; Fat 98% Protein 1% Carbs 1%

Coconut Tea Candy

Servings: 8

Cooking Time: 5 Minutes

Ingredients:

- 2 cups black tea
- 3 tablespoons coconut milk
- Stevia, to taste
- 5 tablespoons gelatine powder

Directions:

1. Take a saucepan and mix the stevia, coconut milk and black tea in it.
2. Cook this mixture to a mixture then add gelatin.
3. After mixing it well enough, pass it through a sieve.
4. Divide the candy mixture into silicone candy molds.
5. Place the candy tray in the refrigerator for 2 hours.
6. Once set, remove the candies from the molds.
7. Serve and enjoy.

Nutrition Info: Calories 136 ;Total Fat 10.7 g ;Saturated Fat 0.5 g ;Cholesterol 4 mg ;Sodium 45 mg ;Total Carbs 1.2 g ;Sugar 1.4 g ;Fiber 0 g ;Protein 0. g

Peppermint Bark

Servings: 12

Cooking Time: 5 Minutes

Ingredients:

- For Dark Chocolate Layer:
- 1/2 teaspoon peppermint extract
- 4 ounces dark chocolate, chopped
- 1/2-ounce cocoa butter
- For White Chocolate Layer:
- 3 tablespoons swerve sweetener
- 1/2 teaspoon peppermint extract, unsweetened
- 2 ounces cocoa butter
- 1/4 cup coconut oil

Directions:

1. Prepare dark chocolate layer and for this, place chocolate and cocoa butter in a heatproof bowl.
2. Microwave the mixture for 45 seconds or more until melted and then stir in peppermint extract.
3. Take a baking sheet, line with parchment paper, then place 24 mini muffin cups and evenly spoon melted chocolate into it, spreading chocolate into the corner.
4. Place muffin cups into the freezer and chill for 30 minutes or more until set and firm.

5. In the meantime, prepare white chocolate layer and for this, place cocoa butter and oil in a heatproof bowl and microwave for 30 seconds or more until melted.

6. Stir well until smooth and then whisk in sweetener and extract until combined.

7. Spread the mixture over dark chocolate layer and freeze for another 15 to 20 minutes or until set.

8. Serve straight away or store in the freezer.

Nutrition Info: Calories: 131 Cal, Carbs: 3.7 g, Fat: 13.8 g, Protein: 0.5 g, Fiber: 1.7 g.

Sugar-free Strawberry And Cream Gummies

Servings: 12-13

Cooking Time: 4-5 Minutes

Ingredients:

- For strawberry layer:
- 1 tablespoon gelatin powder
- 4.5 ounces strawberries
- For cream layer:
- ½ cup coconut milk
- 1 tablespoon gelatin powder
- ½ teaspoon vanilla essence

Directions:

1. For strawberry layer: Add strawberries into a blender and blend until smooth. Transfer into a saucepan. Place the saucepan over low heat.
2. Meanwhile, add gelatin powder into a bowl and add tablespoons of cold water. Whisk until gum like in texture.
3. When the strawberry puree begins to bubble, remove from heat.
4. Add a little of the gelatin mixture at a time into the heated strawberry and whisk well each time. Continue doing this until all the gelatin mixture is added.

5. Divide the mixture into 12 – 13 gummy molds. Fill up to half the molds. Chill until the mix sets. To quicken the process, you can place them in the freezer until they set. Move the gummies into the refrigerator once they set.

6. To make cream layer: Add coconut milk and vanilla essence into a saucepan. Place the saucepan over low heat.

7. Meanwhile, add gelatin powder into a bowl and add 2 tablespoons of cold water. Whisk until gum like in texture.

8. When the coconut milk begins to bubble, remove from heat.

9. Add a little of the gelatin mixture at a time into the heated coconut milk and whisk well each time. Continue doing this until all of the gelatin mixture is added.

10. Divide the mixture into the gummy molds, over the strawberry layer. Chill until they set.

11. Remove from mold and serve.

12. Leftovers can be stored in an airtight container in the refrigerator. These can keep for 4 – 5 days.

Nutrition Info: Per Servings: Calories: kcal, Fat: 0.1 g, Carbohydrates: 0.8 g, Protein: 2 g

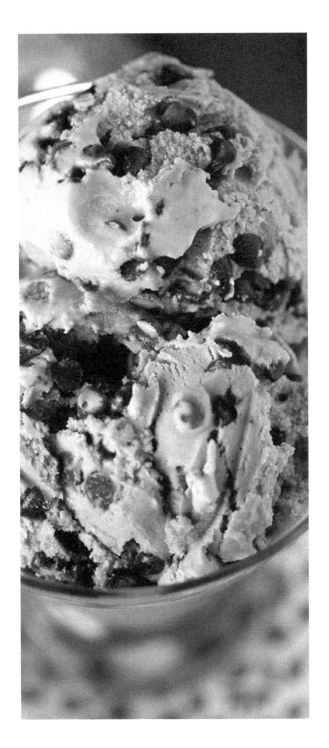

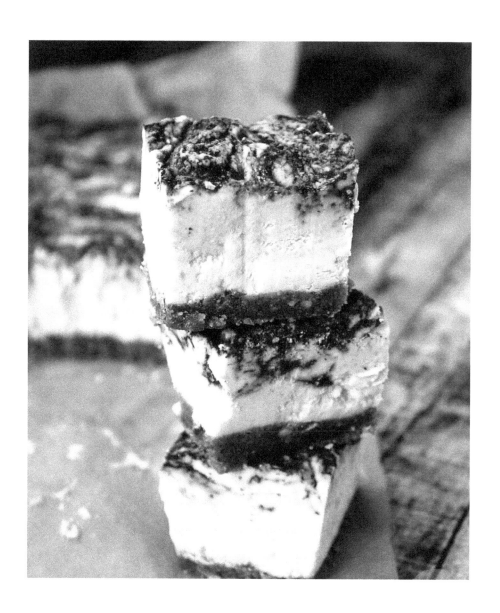

Berry Cheese Candy

Servings: 12

Cooking Time: 5 Minutes

Ingredients:

- 1 cup fresh berries, wash
- 12 cup coconut oil
- 1 12 cup cream cheese, softened
- 1 tbsp vanilla
- 2 tbsp swerve

Directions:

1. Add all ingredients to the blender and blend until smooth and combined.
2. Spoon mixture into small candy molds and refrigerate until set.
3. Serve and enjoy.

Nutrition Info: Per Servings: Net Carbs: 2.3g; Calories: 190; Total Fat: 19.2g; Saturated Fat: 12g Protein: 2.3g; Carbs: 2.7g; Fiber: 0.4g; Sugar: 1g; Fat 90% Protein 5% Carbs 5%

No Bake Keto Coconut Bars

Servings: 10

Cooking Time: 15 Minutes

Ingredients:
- 1 ¼ cups shredded coconut
- 8 tablespoons erythritol
- ½ cup coconut cream
- For topping:
- 20 ounces sugar-free chocolate or chocolate chips

Directions:
1. Add chocolate into a heatproof bowl.
2. Place the bowl in a double boiler. Stir occasionally until the mixture melts. You can also melt it in a small pan over low heat.
3. Meanwhile, add coconut, erythritol and coconut cream into a bowl and mix until small crumbs are formed; it should bind together if pressed.
4. Spoon the coconut mixture into a silicone (rectangle shaped) mold. Spread it evenly and press well into it so that the mix completely fills the mold.
5. Refrigerate for up to 30-40 minutes or until firm.
6. Spoon the melted chocolate over the coconut layer and spread it evenly. Place in the refrigerator for another 30-40 minutes.

7. Cut into 10 equal bars and serve.

8. Leftovers can be stored in an airtight container in the refrigerator. These can keep for 4 – 5 days.

Nutrition Info: Per Servings: Calories: 56.4 kcal, Fat: 5.2 g, Carbohydrates: 11.3 g, Protein: 0.5 g

Turmeric Milk Gummies

Servings: 8

Cooking Time: 5 Minutes

Ingredients:

- ¼ cup of water
- 3 tablespoons gelatine
- 1 cup of coconut milk
- 1 teaspoon turmeric
- ½ teaspoon ginger
- Pinch of freshly ground black pepper
- Pinch of cardamom powder
- Liquid stevia, to taste

Directions:

1. Combine gelatine with water in a saucepan by stirring it well.
2. Heat milk in another saucepan and stir in all the spices on medium heat.
3. After cooking the spiced milk for 5 mins turn off the heat.
4. Add stevia to the milk then pour this mixture into the gelatine mixture.
5. Mix it all well, then pour it into candy molds.
6. Place the molds in the refrigerator for 3 hours.
7. Remove the candies from the molds.

8. Serve and enjoy.

Nutrition Info: Calories 76 ;Total Fat 7.2 g ;Saturated Fat 6.4 g ;Cholesterol 0 mg ;Sodium 8 mg ;Total Carbs 2g ;Sugar 1 g ;Fiber 0.7 g ;Protein 2.2 g

White Chocolate Bark

Servings: 6

Cooking Time: 0 Minute

Ingredients:

- 3/4 cup cacao butter melted
- 1/4 cup cashew butter
- 1/4 cup coconut butter
- 1/4 cup coconut cream
- 3 tbsp liquid coconut nectar
- 2 tsp vanilla essence
- Pinch sea salt

Directions:

1. Blend melted cacao butter with remaining ingredients in a blender until smooth.
2. Spread this mixture in a baking pan into a thin layer.
3. Freeze it for 2 hours.
4. Break into pieces then serve.

Nutrition Info: Per Servings: Calories 193 Total Fat 20 g Saturated Fat 13.2 g Cholesterol 10 mg Total Carbs 2.g Sugar 1 g Fiber 0.7 g Sodium 8 mg Potassium 88 mg Protein 2.2 g

High Protein Green Gummies

Servings: 40-60

Cooking Time: 5 Minutes

Ingredients:

- 1 cup bulletproof collagen
- 2-4 tablespoons xylitol or stevia to taste
- 3 ½ cups freshly made green juice (using greens of your choice, cucumber, lemon juice, lime juice, fresh herbs like mint and basil etc.)

Directions:

1. Add collagen and a cup of green juice into a bowl. Stir and let it sit for a while. In a while it will become thick. Transfer into a saucepan.
2. Add remaining juice and sweetener into the saucepan. Place the saucepan over low heat. Stir frequently until the collagen dissolves completely.
3. Transfer into a small jug with a spout and pour into the gummy molds or into a baking pan lined with parchment paper.
4. Freeze until the gummies are set.
5. Remove from mold and serve. Leftovers can be stored in an airtight container. Cut into small squares if using a pan.
6. Refrigerate until use.

Nutrition Info: Per Servings: Calories: 12.22 kcal, Fat: 0 g, Carbohydrates: 0.12 g, Protein: 2.44 g

Coconut Macadamia Candy

Servings: 14

Cooking Time: 5 Minutes

Ingredients:

- 1 cup macadamia nuts
- 2 tbsp swerve
- 12 cup coconut oil
- 8 drops liquid stevia
- 12 tsp vanilla extract

Directions:

1. Add all ingredients into the blender and blend until smooth.
2. Pour mixture into the silicone candy mold and place in the refrigerator for hours or until candy is hardened.
3. Serve and enjoy.

Nutrition Info: Per Servings: Net Carbs: 0.8g; Calories: 137; Total Fat: 15g; Saturated Fat: 7.9g Protein: 0.8g; Carbs: 1.6g; Fiber: 0.8g; Sugar: 0.5g; Fat 98% Protein 1% Carbs 1%

Raspberry Candy

Servings: 12

Cooking Time: 5 Minutes

Ingredients:

- 12 cup dried raspberries
- 2 oz cacao butter
- 14 cup Swerve
- 12 cup coconut oil

Directions:

1. Melt cacao butter and coconut oil in a saucepan over low heat.
2. Remove saucepan pan from heat.
3. Grind the raspberries in a blender.
4. Add swerve and ground raspberries to the saucepan and stir well.
5. Pour mixture into the silicone candy molds and refrigerate until set.
6. Serve and enjoy.

Nutrition Info: Per Servings: Net Carbs: 0.4g; Calories: 125; Total Fat: 13.8g; Saturated Fat: 11.1g Protein: 0.1g; Carbs: 0.; Fiber: 0.3g; Sugar: 0.2g; Fat 98% Protein 1% Carbs 1%

Chocolate

Servings: 4

Cooking Time: 10 Minutes

Ingredients:

- 1 tsp. vanilla extract, sugar-free
- 4 tbsp. sweetener, confectioner
- 1 cup heavy whipping cream
- 4 tbsp. cocoa powder, unsweetened and sifted
- 1/4 tsp. salt

Directions:

1. Using a food processor on high, whisk the heavy whipping cream for 4 minutes.
2. Combine the sweetener and salt into the mixture. Then add the cocoa powder and vanilla extract until thickened.
3. Spoon the mousse into a pastry bag and pipe into serving dishes.Serve and enjoy!
4. Tricks and Tips:
5. Don´t have a piping bag in your kitchen? You can alternatively use a gallon sized ziplock bag. Just add the whipped cream and cut one corner of the bottom to the size you prefer.

6. If you want a lighter mousse, simply beat 3 egg whites for 4 minutes in a food processor and fold in before spooning into serving dishes.

Nutrition Info: 5 grams ;Net Carbs: 4 grams ;Fat: 26 grams ;Calories: 268

Mocha

Servings: 6

Cooking Time: 2 Hours 25 Minutes

Ingredients:

- 8 oz. mascarpone cheese, softened
- 3 tbsp. sweetener, confectioner
- 1 1/2 cups heavy whipping cream
- 2 tsp. espresso powder, instant
- 1/4 tsp. salt
- 3 tbsp. cocoa powder, unsweetened
- 1 tsp. vanilla extract, sugar-free

Directions:

1. In a food processor on high, whip mascarpone cheese and heavy whipping cream for 6 minutes.
2. Blend the cocoa powder and sweetener and pulse for a minute.
3. Finally add the salt, espresso powder, and vanilla extract until creamy.
4. Spoon the mousse into a pastry bag and pipe into serving cups or dishes.
5. Refrigerate for 2 hours before serving.
6. Tricks and Tips:
7. Don't have a piping bag in your kitchen? You can alternatively use a gallon sized ziplock bag. Just add

the whipped cream and cut one corner of the bottom
to the size you prefer.

Nutrition Info: 4 grams ;Net Carbs: 4 grams ;Fat: 39 grams
;Calories: 3

Caramel Sea Salt

Servings: 1

Cooking Time: 1 Hour

Ingredients:

- 4 tbsp. water
- 1.6 oz. meal replacement shake mix, salted caramel flavor
- 2 tbsp. dark chocolate, unsweetened and chopped
- 1/4 cup heavy whipping cream

Directions:

1. In a food processor on high, whisk the heavy whipping cream for 4 minutes.
2. In a serving cup, mix the water and shake mix until combined. Add the whipped cream.
3. Spoon the mousse into a pastry bag and pipe into a glass or serving dish.
4. Put the glass in the freezer for minutes, stirring the mousse about every 10 minutes.
5. Remove from the freezer and top with chopped chocolate before enjoying.
6. Tricks and Tips:
7. Don´t have a piping bag in your kitchen? You can alternatively use a gallon sized ziplock bag. Just add the whipped cream and cut one corner of the bottom to the size you prefer.

Nutrition Info: 27 grams ;Net Carbs: 5 grams ;Fat: 26 grams ;Calories: 368

Strawberry & Blueberry

Servings: 6

Cooking Time: 10 Minutes

Ingredients:

- 8 oz. mascarpone cheese, softened
- 1/4 cup sweetener, granulated
- 8 oz. strawberries, sliced
- 1 cup heavy whipping cream
- 8 oz. blueberries, whole
- 3/4 tsp. vanilla extract, sugar-free

Directions:

1. Using a food processor set on high, whisk the mascarpone cheese and sweetener for 3 minutes until a smooth consistency.
2. Add in the heavy whipping cream and vanilla extract and continue to whisk for additional minutes.
3. Spoon the mousse into glass cups, layering in the strawberries and blueberries and serve.

Nutrition Info: 3 grams ;Net Carbs: 3 grams ;Fat: 27 grams ;Calories: 260

Avocado

Servings: 6

Cooking Time: 35 Minutes

Ingredients:

- 1 large avocado, shelled
- 3 tsp. lime juice
- 1 tsp. vanilla extract, sugar-free
- 1/4 cup sweetener, confectioner
- 3 tsp. agar agar
- 1 tsp. green tea powder
- 3 tbsp. cold water

Directions:

1. In a regular dish, dispense the water over the agar agar. Allow the mixture soak for 5 minutes before heating in the microwave for minute on the medium/high setting.

2. Using a food processor with an S-blade, stir the avocado, sweetener, green tea powder, and vanilla extract until creamy.

3. Add the agar agar and lime juice to the mousse and stir well.

4. Taste test at this point to add more sweetener to your preference.

5. Spoon the mousse into a pastry bag and pipe into dessert dishes.

6. Cool them for 30 minutes in the refrigerator and serve.

7. Tricks and Tips:

8. If you want variety, you can top the mousse with balsamic vinegar or mixed berries of your choice.

9. Don´t have a piping bag in your kitchen? You can alternatively use a gallon sized ziplock bag. Just add the whipped cream and cut one corner of the bottom to the size you prefer.

Nutrition Info: Calories: 57 ;Net Carbs: 1.3 grams: 1 gram ;Fat: 5 grams

Keto Lemon Popsicles

Servings: 12

Cooking Time: 5 Minutes

Ingredients:

- Zest of 2 lemons, grated
- 4 tablespoons erythritol or to taste
- ½ cup fresh lemon juice
- 4 cups water

Directions:

1. Add zest, erythritol, lemon juice and water into a small pan. Place the pan over medium heat. Stir frequently until the sweetener is dissolved. Turn off the heat and let cool to room temperature.
2. Divide into 1Popsicle molds. Insert popsicle sticks and freeze until firm.
3. To serve: Dip the Popsicle molds in a bowl of warm water for 15 – 20 seconds. The Popsicles will loosen up. Remove from the molds and serve.

Nutrition Info: per Servings: Calories: 26.2 kcal, Fat: 7.6 g, Carbohydrates: 2.2 g, Protein: 0.g

Italian Ricotta Cake

Servings: 8

Cooking Time:1 Hour

Ingredients:

- 2 oz butter, softened
- 1 tsp Stevia/your preferred keto sweetener
- 4 eggs
- 9 oz full fat ricotta
- Juice and zest of 1 lemon
- 1 ½ cups ground almonds
- 2 tsp baking powder
- Pinch of salt

Directions:

1. Preheat the oven to 360 degrees Fahrenheit and line a baking tray with baking paper
2. Beat together the butter and sweetener until soft and creamy
3. Add the eggs to the butter and beat until combined and fluffy
4. Add the ricotta, lemon juice and zest to the bowl and beat until combined and creamy
5. Fold the ground almonds, baking powder and salt into the buttery mixture until just incorporated

6. Pour the batter into your prepared pan and bake for about 45 minutes or until the center of the cake is spongy and bounces back when very gently pressed

7. Leave to cool before slicing and serving!

Nutrition Info: Calories: 199;Fat: 17 grams ;Protein: grams ;Total carbs: 5 grams ;Net carbs: 3 grams

Chocolate French Silk Pie

Servings: 1

Cooking Time: 1 Hour And 10 Minutes

Ingredients:

- For the Crust:
- 1 ¾ tablespoon almond flour
- 1/16 teaspoon salt
- 3 teaspoons Swerve sweetener
- 2 teaspoons cocoa powder
- 3 teaspoons melted butter
- 1/8 teaspoon instant coffee
- For the Filling:
- ½ of a medium avocado
- ¾ tablespoon cocoa powder
- 1/8 teaspoon salt
- 3 tablespoons Swerve sweetener
- 1/2 teaspoon vanilla extract, unsweetened
- 1/4 teaspoon instant coffee
- 1/3 cup coconut milk, full-fat and unsweetened

Directions:

1. Place flour in a bowl, add remaining ingredients and stir until well combined.
2. Take a 4 ½-inch pie dish, line with parchment paper, then spoon in prepared crust mixture and spread and

press down using hands and then with a back of a spoon.

3. Place pie dish into the freezer and let it set.

4. In the meantime, place all the ingredients of filling in a blender and pulse for 1 to 2 minutes at high speed or until smooth.

5. Remove pie pan from the freezer, spoon in prepared filling and smooth the top with a spatula.

6. Return pie pan into the freezer for 1 hour or more until set.

7. Slice and serve.

Nutrition Info: Calories: 394 Cal, Carbs: 13 g, Fat: 37 g, Protein: 9 g, Fiber: g.

Cranberry Curd Tart

Servings: 4

Cooking Time: 25 Minutes

Ingredients:

- Shortbread Tart Crust
- 1 cup blanched superfine almond flour
- 4 tablespoons salted butter
- 1 tablespoon Swerve
- 1 teaspoon vanilla
- Keto Cranberry Curd
- 2-1/2cups cranberries
- ½ cup of water
- 6tablespoons salted butter
- ¼ cup Swerve
- 4 egg yolks
- ½ teaspoon vanilla

Directions:

1. Keto Shortbread Tart Crust
2. Let your oven preheat at 350 degrees F. Grease an 8-inch tart pan.
3. Beat all the ingredients for the crust in an electric mixer to form a smooth dough.
4. Spread this dough in the greased tart pan.
5. Poke some holes in the crust and bake it for 1minutes.

6. Set it aside to cool until filling is ready.

7. Keto Cranberry Curd

8. Boil cranberries with water in a saucepan then reduce the heat to a simmer.

9. Allow it to cool for 5 minutes while smashing the cranberries using a wooden spoon.

10. Pass this berry mixture through a sieve to remove the seeds.

11. This will give 1 cup cranberry puree.

12. Heat this puree in a saucepan then add salt, sweetener, and butter.

13. Mix well then remove it from the heat.

14. Once cooled, whisk in vanilla and egg yolks. Mix well until smooth.

15. Pour this filling in the baked crust.

16. Refrigerate them for 30 minutes.

17. Serve.

Nutrition Info: Per Servings: Calories 215 Total Fat 20 g Saturated Fat 7 g Cholesterol 38 mg Total Carbs 8 g Sugar 1 g Fiber 6 g Sodium 12 mg Potassium 30 mg Protein 5 g

Strawberry Cheesecake Tarts

Servings: 8

Cooking Time: 35 Minutes

Ingredients:

- Crust
- 2 cups almond flour
- 1/4 cup + 1 tbsp granulated Swerve
- 3 oz butter
- Cheesecake filling
- 1 cup cream cheese
- 1/2 cup heavy whipping cream
- 1/4 cup + 1 tbsp confectioners Swerve
- 1/2 tsp sugar-free vanilla essence
- Berry topping
- 1 cup strawberries
- 1 tsp granulated Swerve
- 1/4 tsp sugar-free vanilla essence

Directions:

1. Let your oven preheat at 350 degrees F.
2. Mix almond meal with melted butter and sweetener in a bowl to form a coarse mixture.
3. Grease 6 mini tart pans and divides the crust mixture into the tart pans.

4. Poke some holes in each crust then bake them for 15 minutes.
5. Allow the crust to cool at room temperature.
6. Toss strawberries pieces with vanilla and sweetener in a bowl then spread them in a baking tray.
7. Bake the berries for 20 minutes then allow them to cool.
8. Beat cream cheese with vanilla, and sweetener in an electric mixer until fluffy.
9. Stir in cream and continue beating until creamy.
10. Pass one-half of the strawberries through a sieve to remove all the seeds.
11. Add this puree to the cream cheese mixture and mix gently to make swirls.
12. Divide this mixture into the tart crusts.
13. Refrigerate the tarts for 1 hour.
14. Top them with remaining berries.
15. Serve.

Nutrition Info: Per Servings: Calories 285 Total Fat 27.3 g Saturated Fat 14.5 g Cholesterol 175 mg Total Carbs 3.5 g Sugar 0.4 g Fiber 0.9 g Sodium mg Potassium 83 mg Protein 7.2 g

Chocolate Almond Clusters

Servings: 17

Cooking Time: 50 Minutes

Ingredients:

- 3 ounces dark chocolate, chopped
- 1 cup almonds
- 1 tablespoon erythritol sweetener
- 2 ounces butter, unsalted

Directions:

1. Place chocolate and butter in a heatproof bowl and microwave for 45 seconds or more until melted.
2. Stir in almonds until combined and refrigerate for 10 to 15 minutes or until thick.
3. Then place tablespoons of almond-chocolate mixture onto baking sheets and chill in the freezer for minutes or more until firm.
4. Serve straightaway.

Nutrition Info: Calories: 96 Cal, Carbs: 2 g, Fat: 8.4 g, Protein: 2 g, Fiber: 3.3 g.

Butter Mints

Servings: 4

Cooking Time: 5 Minutes

Ingredients:

- 8 ounces butter
- 1/4 cup raw honey
- 1 teaspoon vanilla essence
- 1/2 teaspoon peppermint extract
- Salt to taste, if using butter, unsalted

Directions:

1. Blend butter with salt, peppermint extract and vanilla essence in a food processor.
2. Spread the parchment paper on a baking tray.
3. Add the butter mixture over baking tray dollop by dollop.
4. Place these butter bites in the freezer for 1 hour.
5. Serve.

Nutrition Info: Per Servings: Calories 91 Total Fat 4.7 g Saturated Fat 0.8 g Cholesterol 11 mg Total Carbs 0 g Sugar 0.2 g Fiber 0.5 g Sodium 43 mg Potassium 181 mg Protein 2 g

Low-carb Brownie Batter Truffles

Servings: 6

Cooking Time: 15 Minutes

Ingredients:

- For brownie truffles:
- ½ cup + 2 tablespoons almond flour
- 3 tablespoons cocoa powder
- ¼ cup butter, melted
- Water, as required
- 3-4 tablespoons Swerve sweetener
- A tiny pinch of salt
- ½ teaspoon vanilla extract
- For chocolate coating:
- ¼ ounce food grade cocoa butter or ½ tablespoon coconut oil
- 1 ½ ounces sugar-free dark chocolate, chopped

Directions:

1. Add all of the dry ingredients into a mixing bowl and stir.
2. Add vanilla and butter and mix until dough is formed. If the dough is not sticking together and is dropping off and falling part as crumbs, add a little water, 1 tablespoon at a time and mix well each time.

3. Form small balls of the dough of about 1 inch diameter. Place on a baking sheet lined with parchment paper.

4. Place the baking sheet in the freezer for an hour or until the balls harden.

5. Meanwhile, add chocolate and cocoa butter into a heatproof bowl. Place the bowl in a double boiler and stir frequently until the mixture melts and is well combined.

6. Dip the truffles in melted chocolate, one at a time and coat each ball well. Pick them up carefully with a fork. Shake to drop off extra melted chocolate. Place each coated ball back on the baking sheet.

7. Place the baking sheet in the freezer for an hour or until the chocolate sets.

8. Serve cold. Leftovers can be stored in an airtight container in the refrigerator. These can last for 5-6 days.

Nutrition Info: Per Servings: Calories: 141.66 kcal, Fat: 14.33 g, Carbohydrates: 3 g, Protein: 3 g

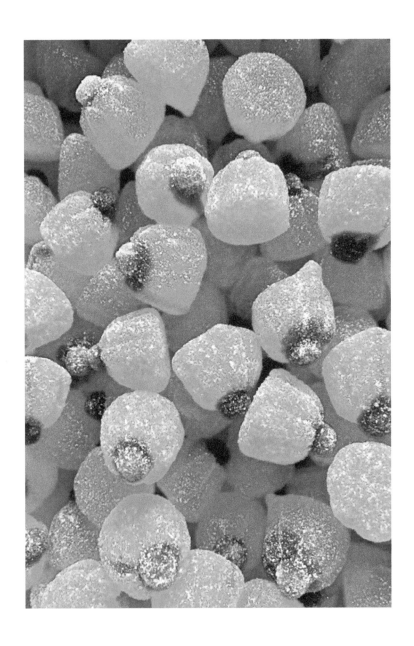

Pumpkin Candy

Servings: 24

Cooking Time: 5 Minutes

Ingredients:

- 12 cup pumpkin
- 13 cup cream cheese, softened
- 12 cup butter, softened
- 1 tbsp pumpkin pie spice
- 12 tbsp vanilla
- 2 packets stevia
- 14 tsp salt

Directions:

1. Add cream cheese and butter in the microwave safe bowl and microwave for 30 seconds. Stir well.
2. Add remaining ingredients and stir until well combined.
3. Pour mixture into the silicone candy mold and refrigerate until set.
4. Serve and enjoy.

Nutrition Info: Per Servings: Net Carbs: 0.7g; Calories: 48 Total Fat: ; Saturated Fat: 3.2g Protein: 0.4g; Carbs: 0.9g; Fiber: 0.2g; Sugar: 0.2g; Fat 93% Protein 3% Carbs 4%

White Chocolate Candy

Servings: 12

Cooking Time: 5 Minutes

Ingredients:

- 12 cup cocoa butter
- 12 tsp vanilla
- 1 scoop vanilla protein powder
- 14 cup erythritol
- Pinch of salt

Directions:

1. Add cocoa butter in a saucepan and heat over medium-low heat until melted.
2. Remove from heat and add remaining ingredients and stir well to combine.
3. Pour mixture into the silicone candy molds and refrigerate until hardened.
4. Serve and enjoy.

Nutrition Info: Per Servings: Net Carbs: 0.1g; Calories: 90; Total Fat: 9.3g; Saturated Fat: 3g Protein: 2.3g; Carbs: 0.1g; Fiber: 0 g; Sugar: 0.1g; Fat 90% Protein 10% Carbs 0%

Mascarpone Cheese Candy

Servings: 10

Cooking Time: 5 Minutes

Ingredients:

- 1 cup mascarpone cheese, softened
- 14 cup pistachios, chopped
- 3 tbsp swerve
- 12 tsp vanilla

Directions:

1. In a small bowl, add swerve, vanilla, and mascarpone and mix together until smooth.
2. Place chopped pistachios in a small shallow dish.
3. Make small balls from cheese mixture and roll in chopped pistachios.
4. Refrigerate for 1 hour.
5. Serve and enjoy.

Nutrition Info: Per Servings: Net Carbs: 1.; Calories: 53 Total Fat: 3.9g; Saturated Fat: 2.1g Protein: 3.1g; Carbs: 1.8g; Fiber: 0.2g; Sugar: 0.2g; Fat 66% Protein 23% Carbs 11%

Peppermint Frost Mints

Servings: 4

Cooking Time: 5 Minutes

Ingredients:

- 1 cup xylitol
- 4 drops peppermint extract

Directions:

1. Cook xylitol in a saucepan over low heat for 5 minutes to melt.
2. Meanwhile, layer a jelly roll pan with wax paper.
3. Allow the xylitol to cool for 10 minutes then add peppermint extract.
4. Mix well then spread this mixture over a baking tray lined with parchment paper.
5. Let it sit overnight to dry the mixture.
6. Break it into bite-sized pieces.
7. Serve.

Nutrition Info: Per Servings: Calories 3Total Fat 0.6 g Saturated Fat 0 g Cholesterol 0 mg Total Carbs 0 g Sugar 0 g Fiber 0 g Sodium 33 mg Potassium 1 mg Protein 9 g

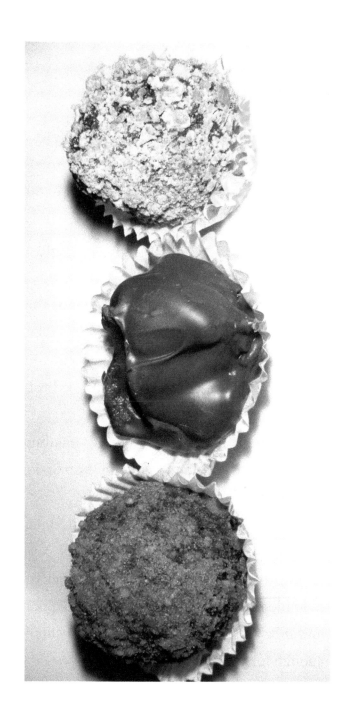

Ultra Decadent Chocolate Truffles

Servings: 20

Cooking Time: 5 Minutes

Ingredients:

- 2 cups coconut cream
- 6-8 tablespoons cocoa powder + extra to dust
- ½ teaspoon kosher salt
- 4-8 tablespoons xylitol or Allulose or any other keto friendly sweetener
- ½ teaspoon espresso powder (optional)
- ½ teaspoon xanthan gum

Directions:

1. Add coconut cream, cocoa, salt, xylitol, espresso powder and salt into a saucepan.
2. Place the saucepan over medium flame. Simultaneously, blend with an immersion blender until smooth.
3. Dust with xanthan gum and continue blending until well incorporated and free from lumps.
4. If you find that the mixture is very thick and you are not able to stir easily, add water, a teaspoon at a time and mix well each time. The mixture should be thick enough for you to shape into truffles so add water only if necessary.

5. Turn off the heat and transfer into a bowl. Cool for a while and cover with cling wrap. Place in the refrigerator until it sets.
6. Make small balls of the mixture of 1-inch diameter.
7. Place some cocoa powder on a plate. Dredge your palms in cocoa powder and roll the balls so that the balls are lightly covered with cocoa. Be quick in doing this or else the balls will start coming back to room temperature. When that happens, they will start losing their shape and you will not be able to dredge. You can also remove a few at a time from the refrigerator and place them back in the refrigerator when done.
8. Transfer into an airtight container. These can last for a week.

Nutrition Info: Per Servings: Calories: 53.1 kcal, Fat: 4.4 g, Carbohydrates: 1.1 g, Protein: 0.8 g

Cinnamon Pecans Candies

Servings: 8

Cooking Time: 15 Minutes

Ingredients:

- 1 cup erythritol
- 1 lb. pecan halves
- 1 egg white
- 1 tablespoon water
- 2 teaspoons cinnamon, ground
- 2 teaspoons ground nutmeg
- 1 teaspoon salt
- Baking spray or butter
- Optional
- 1 teaspoon pumpkin pie spice
- Erythritol, to taste

Directions:

1. Let the oven preheat at 250 degrees F.
2. Combine the dry ingredients in a suitable bowl.
3. Beat egg white with a tablespoon of water until frothy using a mixer.
4. Stir in the dry mixture along with pecans.
5. Mix well to coat all the pecans well.
6. Spread the pecans on a baking sheet.
7. Place this sheet in the preheated oven for 15 minutes.

8. Allow them to cool for a few minutes.

9. Serve.

Nutrition Info: Calories 193 ;Total Fat 20 g ;Saturated Fat 13.2 g ;Cholesterol mg ;Sodium 8 mg ;Total Carbs 2.5 g ;Sugar 1 g ;Fiber 0.7 g ;Protein 2.2 g

Low-carb Strawberry Margarita Gummy Worms

Servings: 12

Cooking Time: 5 Minutes

Ingredients:

- 20 hulled strawberries, fresh or frozen
- 6 tablespoons grass-fed gelatin collagen protein
- 3 ounces fresh lime juice
- 4 ounces silver tequila
- 4 tablespoons powdered erythritol

Directions:

1. Add strawberries and tequila into a blender and blend until smooth.
2. Transfer into a saucepan. Place the saucepan over low heat.
3. Stir in gelatin, lime juice and erythritol. Whisk until gelatin dissolves completely.
4. Whisk frequently. Initially the mixture will be thick. As the mixture heats, it will be more watery.
5. Pour into a cup or small jar with a spout.
6. Pour into gummy worm molds. Chill until it sets.
7. Remove from mold and serve.
8. Leftovers can be stored in an airtight container in the refrigerator. These can keep for 6-7 days.

Nutrition Info: Per Servings: Calories: 6kcal, Fat: 0.16 g,Carbohydrates: 3 g, Protein: 9 g

Cucumber And Lime Sweets

Servings: 4

Cooking Time: 5 Minutes

Ingredients:

- 1 cucumber, peeled
- 15-20 fresh mint leaves
- 1/2 lime juice
- 1.5 tablespoons gelatine powder
- stevia, to taste

Directions:

1. Add stevia, cucumber, mint and lime juices in a blender.
2. Blend these ingredients for a minute.
3. Strain this puree over a saucepan to get its liquid.
4. Cook this liquid to a simmer, then stir in gelatine powder.
5. Once well combined, turn off the heat.
6. Pour this mixture into a silicon candy tray.
7. Place this tray in the refrigerator for 2 hours.
8. Remove the candies from their molds and serve.

Nutrition Info: Calories ;Total Fat 4.7 g ;Saturated Fat 0.8 g ;Cholesterol 11 mg ;Sodium 43 mg ;Total Carbs 0 g ;Sugar 0.2 g ;Fiber 0.5 g ;Protein 2 g

Peanut Butter Cups

Servings: 12

Cooking Time: 1 Hour And 40 Minutes

Ingredients:

- 4 ounces dark chocolate, sugar-free
- 1/3 cup swerve sweetener
- 1/2 teaspoon vanilla extract, unsweetened
- 1/2 cup peanut butter
- 3 ounces cacao butter, chopped
- 1/4 cup butter, unsalted

Directions:

1. Place butter in a small saucepan, place over low heat and stir until smooth.
2. Then stir in sweetener and vanilla until well combined.
3. Line 12 mini muffin tins with cupcake liners and evenly spoon in prepared butter mixture.
4. Place muffin tins into the refrigerator for 1 hour or until firm.
5. Then place chocolate in a small heatproof bowl and microwave for 4seconds or more until melted.
6. Stir until smooth and then spoon this mixture over butter cups, spreading to the edges.
7. Freeze cups more for 15 to 30 minutes or until set.
8. Serve straight away or store in the freezer.

Nutrition Info: Calories: 200 Cal, Carbs: 6.2 g, Fat: 1g, Protein: 2.9 g, Fiber: 3.6 g.

Keto White Chocolate

Servings: 2

Cooking Time: 15-20 Minutes

Ingredients:

- 16 ounces raw cacao butter
- 1 tablespoon dried cranberries (optional)
- 1-2 tablespoons chopped nuts of your choice (optional)
- Cayenne pepper
- 8-10 tablespoons Swerve or powdered erythritol
- 1 teaspoon vanilla extract
- ¾ teaspoon vanilla liquid stevia

Directions:

1. Place a saucepan over low heat. Add cacao butter into it. When it melts, turn off heat. You can also melt it in a double boiler.
2. Add Swerve and whisk well.
3. Line 2 baking sheets with parchment paper. Divide the mixture between the baking sheets. Sprinkle cranberries, cayenne pepper and nuts if using and press lightly into the chocolate mixture.
4. Chill until firm.
5. Break or chop into pieces. Transfer into an airtight container and refrigerate until use.

Nutrition Info: Per Servings: Calories: 193kcal, Fat: 208 g, Carbohydrates: 4 g, Protein: 0 g

Cdb Chocolate Coconut Fat Bombs

Servings: 10 -12

Cooking Time: 1-2 Minutes

Ingredients:

- ¼ cup CBD coconut oil
- ½ tablespoon Brothers Apothecary Wild Rosin Honey
- ¼ cup plain coconut butter (without CBD)

Directions:

1. Add coconut oil, CBD honey and coconut butter into a microwave safe bowl.
2. Microwave on high in increments of 30 seconds. Stir every 30 seconds until the mixture melts and is smooth.
3. Pour into gummy molds. Let it cool for a few minutes.
4. Chill until firm. Remove from mold and serve.
5. Store in an airtight container in the refrigerator. These can keep for a week.

Nutrition Info: Per Servings: Calories: 101 kcal, Fat: 10.25 g, Carbohydrates: 2.25 g, Protein: 0.33 g

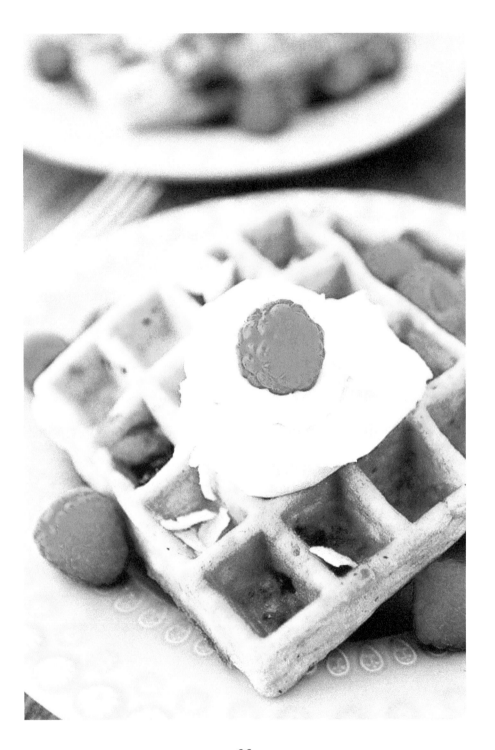

Raspberry Coconut Bark Fat Bombs

Servings: 12

Cooking Time: 1 Hour And 10 Minutes

Ingredients:

- 1/2 cup dried raspberries, frozen
- 1/2 cup shredded coconut, unsweetened
- 1/4 cup powdered swerve sweetener
- 1/2 cup coconut oil
- 1/2 cup coconut butter

Directions:

1. Place berries in a grinder and process at high speed or until a fine powder.
2. Place a saucepan over medium heat, add remaining ingredients, stir well and cook for 3 minutes or more until melted and combined, stirring frequently.
3. Take 8 by 8-inch baking pan, line with parchment paper, then pour half of the prepared mixture in it and spread evenly.
4. Add raspberry powder into the remaining mixture and dollop on mixture in the pan.
5. Swirl with knife and place pan into the refrigerator for 1 hour or more until set and firm.
6. Break into chunks and serve.

Nutrition Info: Calories: 234 Cal, Carbs: 6.5 g, Fat: 23.5 g, Protein: 1.g, Fiber: 4.1 g.

Cocoa Peppermint Fat Bombs

Servings: 8

Cooking Time: 2 Minutes

Ingredients:

- 2 tablespoons coconut oil melted
- 1 tablespoon swerve
- 1/4 teaspoon peppermint essence
- 2 tablespoons cocoa unsweetened

Directions:

1. Mix swerve with peppermint and coconut oil in a suitable bowl.
2. Divide half of this mixture in an ice cube tray.
3. Place the tray in the refrigerator for 1 hour.
4. Add cocoa powder to the reserved mixture and mix well.
5. Pour it over the refrigerated candies.
6. Return the tray to the refrigerator again for 30 minutes.
7. Remove the candies from the tray.
8. Serve.

Nutrition Info: Calories 200 ;Total Fat 21.1 g ;Saturated Fat 15 g ;Cholesterol 14.2 mg ;Sodium 46 mg ;Total Carbs 1.1 g ;Sugar 1.3 g ;Fiber 0.4 g ;Protein 0.4 g

Chocó Almond Candy

Servings: 12

Cooking Time: 5 Minutes

Ingredients:

- 3 tbsp pure cocoa nibs
- 14 cup almonds, crushed
- 1 cup unsweetened cocoa powder
- 1 tsp vanilla
- 8 tbsp coconut oil

Directions:

1. Melt coconut oil in a saucepan over low heat.
2. Remove saucepan from heat.
3. Add remaining ingredients and stir well to combine.
4. Pour mixture into the silicone candy mold and refrigerate until hardened.
5. Serve and enjoy.

Nutrition Info: Per Servings: Net Carbs: 2g; Calories: 11Total Fat: 12g; Saturated Fat: 9.1g Protein: 2g; Carbs: 4.9g; Fiber: 2.9g; Sugar: 0.3g; Fat 90% Protein 5% Carbs 5%

Peanut Butter Coconut Candy

Servings: 20

Cooking Time: 5 Minutes

Ingredients:

- 1 tsp vanilla
- 2 tbsp coconut milk
- 1 12 tbsp coconut oil
- 14 cup peanut butter
- 1 cup of cocoa butter
- 10 drops stevia
- 14 tsp sea salt

Directions:

1. Add all ingredients except stevia and sea salt in a saucepan and heat over low heat just until melted.
2. Stir in stevia and sea salt.
3. Pour mixture into the silicone candy molds and refrigerate until set.
4. Serve and enjoy.

Nutrition Info: Per Servings: Net Carbs: 0.6g; Calories: 128; Total Fat: 14.2g; Saturated Fat: 7.9g Protein: 0.8g; Carbs: 0.8g; Fiber: 0.2g; Sugar: 0.4g; Fat 98% Protein 1% Carbs 1%

Lemon Drop Gummies

Servings: 12

Cooking Time: 0 Minute

Ingredients:

- 1/4 cup fresh lemon juice
- 1 tablespoon water
- 2 tablespoons gelatine powder
- 2 tablespoons erythritol or stevia, to taste

Directions:

1. Let the lemon juice and water warm up in a saucepan.
2. Gradually stir in erythritol and gelatine powder. Mix well.
3. Divide the mixture into silicone molds.
4. Refrigerate them for 2 hours until set.
5. Serve after removing them from the molds.

Nutrition Info: Per Servings: Calories 139 Total Fat 4.g Saturated Fat 0.5 g Cholesterol 1.2 mg Total Carbs 7.5 g Sugar 6.3 g Fiber 0.6 g Sodium 83 mg Potassium 113 mg Protein 3.8 g

Peppermint Candies

Servings: 12

Cooking Time: 3 Minutes

Ingredients:

- 1/2 cup coconut butter
- 1/4 cup unsweetened coconut, shredded
- 2 tablespoons coconut oil
- 1 teaspoon peppermint extract
- Erythritol to taste
- 4 oz. sugar-free dark chocolate
- 4 tablespoons coconut oil

Directions:

1. First, melt the coconut butter in a saucepan.
2. Add tbsp coconut oil, peppermint, stevia and coconut shreds.
3. Cook this mixture until well heated and mixed.
4. Let it cool for 5 mins then divide it into small muffin cups.
5. Place the muffin cups in the refrigerator for 1 hour.
6. Meanwhile, melt the dark chocolate and 4 tbsp coconut oil in a microwave.
7. Pour this mixture into the muffin cups.
8. Let them again cool in the refrigerator for 1 hour.
9. Remove the candies from the cups and enjoy.

Nutrition Info: Calories 139 ;Total Fat 4.6 g ;Saturated Fat 0.5 g ;Cholesterol 1.2 mg ;Sodium 83 mg ;Total Carbs 7.5 g ;Sugar 6.3 g ;Fiber 0.6 g ;Protein 3.8 g

Strawberry Candy

Servings: 12

Cooking Time: 10 Minutes

Ingredients:

- 3 fresh strawberries
- 12 cup butter, softened
- 8 oz cream cheese, softened
- 12 tsp vanilla
- 34 cup Swerve

Directions:

1. Add all ingredients into the food processor and process until smooth.
2. Pour mixture into the silicone candy mold and place in the refrigerator for hours or until candy is hardened.
3. Serve and enjoy.

Nutrition Info: Per Servings: Net Carbs: 0.8g; Calories: 136 Total Fat: 13g; Saturated Fat: 9g Protein: 1.5g; Carbs: 0.9g; Fiber: 0.1g; Sugar: 0.2g; Fat 94% Protein 4% Carbs 2%

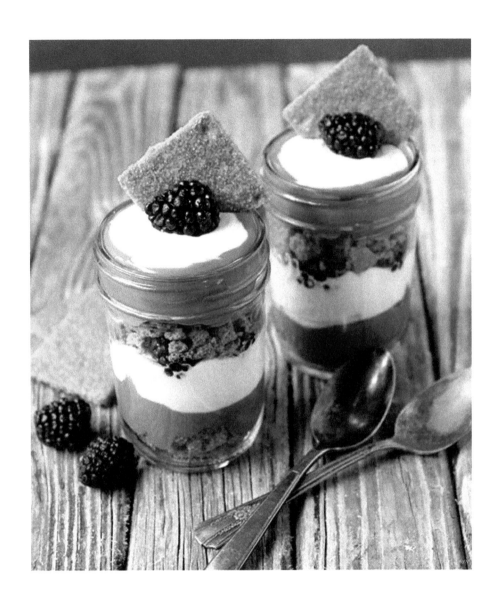

Blackberry Candy

Servings: 8

Cooking Time: 5 Minutes

Ingredients:

- 12 cup fresh blackberries
- 14 cup cashew butter
- 1 tbsp fresh lemon juice
- 12 cup coconut oil
- 12 cup unsweetened coconut milk

Directions:

1. Heat cashew butter, coconut oil, and coconut milk in a pan over medium-low heat, until just warm.
2. Transfer cashew butter mixture to the blender along with remaining ingredients and blend until smooth.
3. Pour mixture into the silicone candy mold and refrigerate until set.
4. Serve and enjoy.

Nutrition Info: Per Servings: Net Carbs: 2.9g; Calories: 203; Total Fat: 21.2g; Saturated Fat: 18g Protein: 1.9g; Carbs: 3.9g; Fiber: 1g; Sugar: 1g; Fat 92% Protein 3% Carbs 5%

3-way Keto Fudge

Servings: 25-28

Cooking Time: 10 Minutes

Ingredients:

- Keto fudge base with vanilla flavor:
- ½ cup coconut butter
- 4-8 tablespoons collagen peptides
- 1/8 teaspoon salt
- 20 drops liquid stevia or monk fruit sweetener to taste
- 1 teaspoon vanilla extract
- 4-6 tablespoons Brain Octane oil
- For chocolate fudge additions:
- 2-4 teaspoons cacao powder
- 2-4 drops liquid stevia or monk fruit sweetener to taste
- 1 teaspoon ground cinnamon
- For turmeric fudge additions:
- 2-4 drops liquid stevia or monk fruit sweetener to taste (optional)
- 1-2 teaspoons turmeric powder

Directions:

1. For vanilla fudge base: Add coconut butter, salt, stevia, 4 tablespoons Brain octane oil and vanilla into a saucepan.

2. Place the saucepan over medium-low heat. Stir frequently until the mixture melts and is well combined. Turn off the heat.

3. Add 4 tablespoons collagen peptides and stir until well incorporated. If the mixture is very watery, add more collagen, 1 tablespoon at a time and stir well each time. If the mixture is very thick, add 1-2 tablespoons Brain octane oil.

4. For vanilla fudge: After step 3, spoon into molds and freeze until firm.

5. For chocolate fudge: Add cacao, sweetener and cinnamon in step 3. Mix well and spoon into molds. Freeze until firm.

6. For turmeric fudge: Add turmeric and sweetener in step 3. Mix well and spoon into molds. Freeze until firm.

7. Remove from molds and place in an airtight container. Refrigerate until use.

Nutrition Info: Per Servings: Calories: 72. kcal, Fat: 6.32 g, Carbohydrates: 1.28 g, Protein: 2.4 g